The Bowl of Sacred Power
15 Spiritual Energies of Menstruation

This book is packed full of information for all females, from young girls (the power of their first blood) to mature women (the wisdom of the crone). In it you will discover:

- The sacredness of womanhood, her powerful connection to the moon cycle honored by cultures and rituals throughout history
- The mystery of female quantum entanglement, her powerful dreams and intuition
- Ixchel the goddess of fertility, the wisdom of the crone
- Egg and womb consciousness
- Scientific research of menstrual blood stem cells
- Ancient women's wisdom of the yoni steam using healing herbs
- Prayers and imagery honoring the divine feminine

Pick up this fast read packed full of information today. Learn and share the wisdom of every woman's birthright.

Your Amazing Itty Bitty® Bowl of Sacred Power Book

15 Spiritual Energies of Menstruation

Rhona Jordan
C.GIt., C.CHt.

Published by Itty Bitty® Publishing
A subsidiary of S & P Productions, Inc.

Copyright © 2019 **Rhona Jordan, C.GIt., C.CHt.**

All rights reserved. No part of this book may be reproduced or transmitted in any form or by any means, electronic or mechanical, including photocopying, recording or by any information storage and retrieval system, without written permission of the publisher, except for inclusion of brief quotations in a review.

Printed in the United States of America

Itty Bitty Publishing
311 Main Street, Suite D
El Segundo, CA 90245
(310) 640-8885

ISBN: 978-1-950326-27-3

Photograph of Rhona Jordan courtesy of Prasad Photographer.

Dedication

I dedicate this especially with deep knowing and heart to heart, egg to egg connection to my beautiful daughter, Heather, my extraordinary granddaughter, Lauren and all girls, mothers, aunts, sisters, daughters and granddaughters.

To my husband, son-in-law, our grandsons. To all boys and men, fathers, grandfathers, uncles and sons who respect and lovingly support the bowl of sacred power held by girls and women.

A warm thank you to Sherine Aubert, PT, DPT, PRPC, whose informative lecture describing the "bowl" inspired the title for this book. Dr. Sherine, I love working beside you at Sarton Physical Therapy clinic in Tustin, California.

Stop by our Itty Bitty® website to find to find more information about women and their sacred energies at:

www.IttyBittyPublishing.com

Or visit Rhona Jordan at

www.RhonaImagery.com

Table of Contents

Introduction
Spiritual 1. The Bowl of Sacred Power
Spiritual 2. The Power of First Blood, the Period
Spiritual 3. The Egg and Alchemy
Spiritual 4. Rest, Dream, Pineal Gland, Prophecy, Consciousness
Spiritual 5. Quantum Entanglement
Spiritual 6. The Crone, Wisdom Keeper
Spiritual 7. Bowl of Sacred Power Chakras
Spiritual 8. Stem Cell Menstrual Blood Research
Spiritual 9. The Powers of Smudge, Smoke, and Steam
Spiritual 10. Cultural History and Rituals
Spiritual 11. Yoni Steam and Herbs
Spiritual 12. Ixchel, Goddess of Fertility, Cozumel, Mexico
Spiritual 13. The Jaguar, Consciousness Shift
Spiritual 14. Divine Feminine
Spiritual 15. Prayers and Imagery

Introduction

The blessing of the feminine womb was first celebrated thousands of years ago in ancient myths and religions throughout the world which honored the sacred regenerative properties of the "flowering" of our wombs. Menstrual blood was the most sacred substance on earth and now it is being rediscovered for the incredible healing abilities of its stem cells.

In many cultures, legends have been passed down about the menstrual powers of female shamans being stolen by male gods. It is well documented that for the last 1,000 years, the rise of male dominated patriarchy ideologies barred all celebration and even Christian rites of the menstrual mysteries.

Research scientists in the United States, India, China, Russia and several other top international locations are working with menstrual blood stem cells and the research is indicating their incredible regenerative healing abilities.

In the writings of the ancients, the moon cycle and woman's cycle were the same. Menstruation is called moon time and the

Crone, when you hold your blood, is called moon pause or menopause.

Long ago before big pharma, women knew how to self-care by steaming different herbs for vaginal health, called the yoni steam. This self-treatment is now returning and being used by modern women.

Women's quantum entanglement, intuition and dreams have always been powerful. In ancient times, the dreams they had during their menstrual or moon times were profound and they shared the insights from these dreams with the village. Their expanded awareness served the village. When connected to the intuition of their menstrual time, today's women have those same powerful abilities.

Spiritual Energy 1
The Bowl of Sacred Power

The bowl holds a woman's sacred power, her sacred energy. It is the source of female creative expression, magic and intuition.

1. In a female's body, the sacred sacrum in the back, pubis bone in the front, and hipbones on each side form a protected bowl.
2. The bowl connects the lower and upper parts of the body.
3. The bowl's location is the center of the body's gravity.
4. The sacred vaginal gateway is the portal to bring in a spiritual entity from another dimension to this dimension.
5. The base of the bowl contains the sacred "V".

The Bowl and Menstruation

The term menstruation comes from the Latin word *mensis,* which means month. It is also related to the Greek word *mene,* which means moon.

- The magnetic pull of the moon and earth affect the primordial fluid tides in the female body.
- Females have a sacred alliance with the mysteries of the universe and quantum entanglement.
- There is an alchemy of the egg, fetus, spirit, baby and birth.
- There is a gut-brain tissue and instinct connection.
- Deep instincts reside here that perhaps have not yet evolved to self-doubt like the head and heart have.
- We say things like, "I feel it in my gut" and "my gut tells me to".
- It is tied strongly to emotions: survival, reproduction, digestion, assimilation and elimination.

Spiritual Energy 2
The Power of First Blood, The Period

Looking at your first blood changes everything. It is an awakening to the scared event in spirit, body, and mind. Effects of the first blood:

1. First blood is the alchemy transformation: the butterfly that leaves the safe cocoon of childhood and morphs into girlhood, then womanhood.
2. Seemingly overnight, a young girl becomes a blossoming, young woman as she skips and dances with her bowl of sacred power.
3. This is a sacred time to join girls and women in the red lodge for dreaming.
4. The girl's life path changes from being a child to becoming a grown up.
5. A transformation occurs in the body and in the mind.
6. There is an awakening of the sacredness within you.
7. Behind the eyes, deep within the brain, resides the pineal gland and it is waiting for the chemical menstrual signal to stimulate awareness beyond the three dimensional known world.

Why is it Called The Period?

- Menstruation happens periodically, as in a cycle, or in a period of time.
- The period is a quantum, atomic and sub atomic energy expression.
- The period represents great unmatched power.
- The period is unbounded, unlimited potential.
- A period or circle used in astrology represents the planet earth.
- The period is condensed energy.
- The period is the void, the creation.

Spiritual Energy 3
The Egg and Alchemy

The day your mother was born all of her eggs were intact and you were one of her eggs and were born with her. Every emotion she ever experienced created chemicals, and these molecules of emotion bathed you, the egg, leaving an imprint of her experiences.

1. Hormones affect tissue and emotions, reminding you of the opportunity to care for self.
2. Everything in the universe is energy changing form, including your eggs.
3. You are energy, frequency and vibration.
4. All frequency carries information.
5. Choices and actions are energy that can support or harm.
6. The environment affects the egg.
7. Think of all the grandmothers before your mother.
8. Think of you as the egg.
9. Think of the eggs you are carrying.
10. The words you say are frequency, energy, and vibration and affect the egg.
11. Protect and care for your eggs; with your thoughts, actions and choices.

More About The Egg

There are benefits from acknowledging and respecting the connection between the universe, your body and your eggs.

- Make a conscious choice of what you put into your body since it becomes your flesh.
- Do not harm your body; protect your body; protect your eggs.
- You are the powerful link in the chain of egg events for future children and their children and their children's children.

Spiritual Energy 4
Rest, Dream, Pineal Gland, Prophecy, Consciousness

The red tent represents a sacred place for the female during her period to relax and honor her womb journey as the bowl is emptying and creating space to re-fill. This is a time of great spiritual opportunity.

1. Hormones affect tissue and emotions, reminding you of the opportunity to care for self.
2. Give yourself the gift of this time to be alone for reflection and dreaming.
3. Resting the body is honoring the body and the bowl of sacred power.
4. The bloat in the belly is the palatable sign of the moon growing within.
5. Honor the clean sacred blood, the powerful, regenerating stem cells.
6. Nurture and love the self unconditionally; respect the self.
7. Looking into the light of the moon stimulates a primal ancient knowing.
8. Honor your sacred moon time.
9. Embrace the awareness of your bowl of sacred power.
10. Trust your intuitions; trust your dreams.
11. Be aware of expanded consciousness.

The Pineal Gland

Womb centered awareness and controlled breathing stimulate the pineal gland which releases melatonin and other chemicals, thus altering the brain for stronger intuition, cosmic connection, and higher states of consciousness.

- The pineal gland is the key to open the portal bringing information and enlightenment.
- The pineal gland produces melatonin, a serotonin-derived hormone which modulates sleep patterns and seasonal, celestial cycles.
- It looks like a pine cone and is centered between the two hemispheres of the brain.
- When this gland is stimulated, we can enter other dimensions, other realities.

Spiritual Energy 5
Quantum Entanglement

Quantum entanglement means we are all connected. Quantum theory asserts that the particles of energy/matter become correlated and interact with each other. Entanglement is a real phenomenon. Dr. Albert Einstein called it "spooky action at a distance". We, as women, are very connected to the moon and to the earth.

1. The earth mother is alive, and you live on her fertile back.
2. The earth is considered feminine.
3. The moon is considered feminine.
4. Women who work together often have their periods at the same time.
5. Best girlfriends often have their periods at the same time.
6. Families with multiple girls often bleed at the same time.

Our Powerful Connection to the Moon

The moon has a powerful magnetic pull on the fluid tides within women's bodies and the tides of the oceans.

- The moon cycle is 29 days.
- The average menstrual cycle is 28 days.
- Many women have their periods during the dark moon.
- The moon phases influence the hormonal cycles of vaginal fluids, basal body temperature and blood.

Long ago, before we lived in concrete cities and had artificial light, the light of the moon and our connection to the earth triggered our natural rhythms and cycles.

- Look at the moon and allow the light to enter your eyes.
- Renew your connection, recalibrate your moon cycle to its natural rhythm of nature.
- Primordial lunar cycles are your natural inheritance.

Spiritual Energy 6
The Crone, Wisdom Keeper

We are here for seasons. Winter comes after the seasons of spring, summer and fall and with it the energy of the crone, a woman of power, filled with life experiences. Even though we no longer bleed, we are still connected to each woman and to the pull of the moon. We may have had a hysterectomy earlier in life, however, on an energy level, the uterus is still intact and we can feel the energies of the sacred womb.

1. We celebrate our Moon Pause (menopause), when blood stops, also known as holding the blood.
2. This is a continuation of the natural cycles, rhythms and the alchemy of energy changing form.
3. It is a time to adjust to changes in our body, skin, hair, sleep patterns, energy, memory, illness and aches; all that accrues during the winter, the last season of life.
4. There is a celebration of entering the grandmother lodge which holds the mystery and wisdom of the cosmos.
5. Grandmother wisdom embraces the role of the healer, sage, wisdom keeper, egg and womb guardian.

Alchemy and Gently Stepping Into a New Normal

The crone celebrates this new normal, free to explore who she is becoming by reinventing self. She is flexible in spirit and mind.

- Once you were the void, the egg, the embryo, the fetus, the baby.
- You are energy and energy always changes form.
- You are still changing form as the crone.
- The crone uses all the skills and tools gathered during the life seasons.
- The crone is excited to learn new skills, gather new tools, taste new foods, read, write, explore, travel, share stories, teach, and play.
- The crone is deeply aware of her spirituality and connection to all that is.

Spiritual Energy 7
Bowl of Sacred Power Chakras

Chakra is a Sanskrit word that describes a wheel or disk that corresponds to massive nerve centers in the body. A chakra is the junction point between consciousness and the physical body. Seven thousand years of Vedic ancient sacred text handed down through wisdom teachers for generations teaches about the primordial chakras.

1. There are seven main chakras in the human body.
2. Each main chakra has a color, frequency, and vibrational sound,
3. Chakras 4 – 7: connect matter with spirit;
4. Chakras 1 through 3: survival and reproduction
5. Chakra 1 and 2 are associated with the bowl.
6. The first chakra located at the perineum is the foundation, the base of the energetic spine
7. The first chakra governs our impulses and supports the upper six chakras.
8. Some consider the first chakra to be the most important one.

The Bowl of Sacred Power Chakras

The first two chakras relate to a woman's bowl of sacred power.

- **1st Chakra – Root**
- Located at the perineum, the base of the pelvic floor.
- Musical note C, color red, sound is LAM.
- Survival, sex reproduction, rectum, tailbone, bladder, colon, first 3 vertebrae
- **2nd Chakra – Sacral**
- Located 2 inches below the navel.
- Musical note D, color orange, sound is VAM.
- Creativity, expression, womb, blood sugar, spleen, ovaries, urinary tract, kidney, adrenals, reproduction system

Spiritual Energy 8
Stem Cell Menstrual Blood Research

Scientific research of stem cells shows that there are remarkable uses for them.

1. Menstrual blood stem cells are powerful and abundant, non-controversial and easily collected.
2. Stromal stem cells are in the endometrial tissues of the uterus and shed each month; they are multi-potency.
3. Menstrual blood contains precursor cells used for cardiac stem cell therapeutic material.
4. One day in the future women could use their menstrual blood for their own treatments; doing so would overcome the major problems of immune system rejection.

More About Stem Cells

Other properties of stem cells are:

- Stem cells are capable of self-renewal,
- Stem cells produce new blood, immune cells, red and white blood cells, platelets.
- Stem cells can be induced to become any desired cell type to regenerate damaged tissue or organs.
- Stem cells are engineered into new skin for burn victims.
- Stem cells create blood vessels for cardiovascular or vascular disease.
- Stem cells will be able to treat brain disease, Alzheimer's or Parkinson's.

Spiritual Energy 9
The Powers of Smudge, Smoke, and Steam

Your body and the earth send out electromagnetic energy. Together they form the electromagnetic field. This field is affected by smoke, steam, incense, and herbs that release negative ions into the atmosphere. This release allows your energy and the energy field around you to be uplifted by the herbs' higher frequency and vibration.

1. The ancient wisdom and traditions of smudging, boiling and steaming or burning herbs, incense and resins are used for the body's healing, spiritual and emotional needs.
2. Scientific study of smoke shows it can be a powerful antiseptic purifying the air of 94% of harmful bacteria up to 24 hours.
3. Sage and sweetgrass are burned to clean or smudge the body, the space around the body, a room or area from negativity or when preparing the V-steam.

The Vaginal Steam – A Specific Example

Women practiced self-care centuries before there were medical doctors, hospitals and clinics. The vaginal steam, also known as the yoni steam, is one example of this self-care.

- Ancient cultures used herb-infused steam for detoxification, soothing, recalibrating the cycle, starting or ending menstrual flow, to help with fertilization or to miscarry and to heal some vaginal conditions.
- The vaginal mucus membranes, blood, and skin absorb this ancient natural remedy for healing the vagina, womb, reproductive tract, soothing hemorrhoids, balancing hormones, relieving headaches and fatigue, helping with infertility, and for better skin appearance.
- Modern medical science has not proved or disproved vaginal steaming benefits.
- As with most ancient and natural home remedies, there is no accepted medical science or medical guidelines.
- Consult with your alternative healthcare professional, Ayurvedic doctor or Chinese Acupuncturist before experiencing the vaginal steam.
- See Chapter 11 for more information.

Spiritual Energy 10
Cultural History and Rituals

The cultural history and rituals surrounding the womb and menstruation from ancient times are worldwide.

1. The Holy Grail, in its true original essence, is the womb.
2. The Maoris in New Zealand feel human menstrual womb blood assumes human form and the human soul.
3. Africans said menstrual blood is "congealed to fashion a man".
4. Hindu believe as the Great Mother creates, her substances become thickened and form a curd or clot. This was the way she gave birth to the cosmos and women employ the same method on a smaller scale.
5. South American Indians said "all mankind was made of moon blood in the beginning".
6. Ancient Mesopotamia believed the Great Goddess Ninhursag made mankind out of clay infused with her "blood of life".

More Cultural History and Rituals

- Egyptian pharaohs became divine by ingesting "the blood of Isis", an ambrosia called SA. Its hieroglyphic sign was the same as the sign of the vulva, a yonic loop like the one on the ankh or Cross of Life. Painted red, this loop signified the female vagina, the Gate of Heaven.
- Persia had the same elixir of immortality called Amritas sometimes called the Milk of the Mother Goddess; it is always associated with the moon and blood.
- Celtic kings became gods by drinking the "red mead" dispensed by the Fairy Queen Mab, whose name was formerly Medhbh or mead. A Celtic name for this fluid was dergflaith, meaning red ale or red sovereignty. In Celtic Britain, to be stained with red mead is to be chosen by the goddess as king.
- Greek mystics spoke of the Apha river (meaning the beginning) also named Styx. The river wound seven times through the earth's interior and emerged at a yonic shrine near the city of Clitor (Greek Kleitoris) sacred to the Great Mother. Styx was the blood-stream from the earth's vagina.

Spiritual Energy 11
Yoni Steam and Herbs

Yoni is a Sanskrit word for vagina/womb. The yoni steam is also known as vaginal steam, V-steam, and peri-steam hydrotherapy. Yoni steam has been found in ancient cultures and literature from China, Africa, Korea, Egypt, Greece, India, South America, Japan, Mexico and the Phillippines. Herbs are the key and steaming is the vehicle for carrying them into your body through the sensitive mucous membranes and the skin. There are many benefits of vaginal steaming varying with the different herbs used.

1. Promotes overall vaginal health.
2. Cares for the sacred womb space.
3. Prepares the body for the first blood.
4. Eases cramps and boosts fertility.
5. A pre- and post-child birth cleanse.
6. Provides relief for pre- and post-menopausal symptoms.
7. Aids recovery after vaginal or womb surgery reducing swelling and disinfecting wounds.
8. Improves circulation, softens scar tissue and supports general skin care.
9. Supports restful, restorative sleep.
10. Can be used before the first period through the crone years.

A Yoni Steam at Home

The yoni steam is available at many alternative clinics and skin care communities, or you may prefer to experience it in your own home. Prepackaged yoni steam herbs, yoni steam stools and chairs can all be purchased on the internet.

- Herbs are very powerful; know the herbs being used and why they were selected for your body; some encourage a miscarriage or make symptoms worse.
- Boil the selected herbs for a few minutes;
- Place the hot herb pot on the floor (use a hot plate if needed) under the yoni stool.
- Always test steam temperature with the palm of your hand by placing it at the opening of the stool to make sure it is comfortable and not too hot.
- When the steam is a comfortable and soothing temperature, sit and wrap a large beach towel around you to keep the steam contained; either wrapping it from just below your neck or from the waist down.
- Enjoy the yoni steam for 30 minutes maximum while you meditate, read something inspirational; honor the sacredness of you and your bowl of sacred power, being a woman.
- Use the herbs only once and then return them to the earth, to the garden or yard.

Spiritual Energy 12
Ixchel, Goddess of Fertility
Cozumel, Mexico

Two thousand years ago, Ixchel (pronounced Ishchel) was the most important Mayan Goddess, and none matched her power and beauty. She represented earth's fertility, earth cycles: moon, planting, the harvest and the rain. The entire island of Cozumel (Mexico) was her domain.

- Ixchel's temple site was used for worship, praying for fertility, spiritual and physical healing and birthing.
- There is a present-day shrine to Ixchel in the San Gervasio Ruins on Transversal Road in Cozumel, Mexico, accessible by a short ferry ride.
- Village healers traveled to the island to learn skills from the priestesses and return to better serve their people.
- The Goddess protected the pilgrims who visited her sacred island.
- Ixchel was the wife of the Sun God Ak Kin who became jealous and abusive so she took the form of a jaguar and became invisible whenever he searched for her.
- Ixchel encourages all women to be assertive and to take one's self away from emotional or physical violence.

More About the Mayan Goddess Ixchel

- Ixchel's name is Chak Chet in Mayan hieroglyphics meaning large rainbow.
- Ixchel is known by many names: Jaguar Goddess, Moon/Lunar Goddess, Fertility Goddess, Goddess of Textile Arts, Goddess of Medicine, Rainbow Woman.
- Ixchel is represented by a beautiful young woman holding a rabbit (fertility), an old woman knitting on a waist loom (weaving the community), sometimes with the clawed feet of the jaguar, the wisdom snake on her head, pouring an upside-down jug of water to the earth.
- Ixchel temple guardians were high priestesses, wise women, teachers, healers, and midwives.
- Twice in a Mayan woman's lifetime she made the dangerous canoe journey to Cozumel where she was attended by the priestesses as she prayed to Ixchel for fertility, safe delivery and health.
- The initial voyage was made by a young girl with her mother shortly after her first period.
- The second voyage was made once she took her own daughter to celebrate the daughter's first period.
- Vaginal steam was an important ritual for health and the steam ruins are still visible today at the temple site.

Spiritual Energy 13
The Jaguar, Consciousness Shift

Here is a story of a powerful consciousness shift. In March 1994, I received an unexpected call and within 24 hours arrived in the village of Palenque, Mexico, to see the pyramid tomb of Pakal, the Mayan King ruler who died over 1,500 years ago. He is still in his carved sarcophagus that appears to show him in a modern-day space ship. Several times I explored Pakal's tomb, and each time I had a fearful and mystical experience.

1. I was staying in the jungle with Elke, a shaman, a healer woman, in her home a mile from the pyramid.
2. Elke's home had three levels of cement floors with no walls, hammocks for sleeping and a small outdoor bathroom.
3. No one sleeps on the first floor due to the animals and dogs that roomed the night.
4. Elke took me to visit her friend in the village of Chiapas on a mountaintop plateau not knowing that less than two months before there was a civil war in Chiapas and many people were killed.
5. Elke's friend, a Mayan dancer and owner of a small restaurant, quickly hid us in her home; there was no safe place.

The Journey Continues

- Every night I had more frightening dreams and mystical experiences. After the 4th night I decided to return home.
- When saying goodbye, Elke gifted me a white cotton ceremonial dress she had sewn; the front is a hand painted Jaguar.
- The jaguar is a divine figure, the possessor of knowledge and stands for power, fertility, virtue and integrity.
- Life as I knew it had changed forever.
- This story illustrates how my bowl of sacred power and the pineal gland were activated and how they opened the doorway for experiences beyond the 3rd dimension to embrace and integrate the gifts I was given at birth.
- This Mayan adventure, the Jaguar, was the start of taking my bowl of sacred power on many Indiana Jones-type adventures, all of them mystical, powerful, consciousness shifts.
- Writing about the Goddess Ixchel, reminded me of the power of shape shifting, being unseen, having keen vision, and pure power.
- Every morning during meditation, I speak out loud to the Jaguar spirit and feel the presence of the Jaguar walking beside me.

Spiritual Energy 14
Divine Feminine

The term "divine feminine" refers to the goddess in all traditions since the beginning of time and represents all nurturing and healing. Characteristics of the divine feminine are:

1. Woman is mystical and mysterious.
2. Woman has the womb, primordial space.
3. Woman carries the eggs, the future.
4. Woman's womb is the cosmic void, the portal that brings a being from one dimension into another realm.
5. Woman loves deeply.
6. Woman protects.
7. A woman is formidable, a warrior.
8. Woman nourishes.
9. Woman is a story teller and teacher.
10. Woman bonds the family together.
11. Woman is a natural healer.
12. Woman gives birth.
13. Woman sustains life with her body.
14. Woman is wise, a sage.
15. Woman is a friend, mother, daughter, aunt, sister, goddess.
16. Woman is powerful beyond measure.
17. Women's stem cells are life for healing and considered the Holy Grail.

More About the Divine Feminine

- Woman awakens the dream.
- Woman's intuition is from a direct download for cosmic information.
- Woman is the messenger connected to earth's frequency.
- Woman's earth steps are guided in true power, balance and harmony.
- Woman's primordial tides ebb and flow, cycling with the moon.

Spiritual Energy 15
Prayers and Imagery

Goddess of the womb, cast off all impurities and retain that which is pure.
- Taoist Prayer

Water is my blood
Earth is my body
Air is my breath
Fire is my spirit
- Native Prayer

1. Imagine a sacred place where women gather and celebrate their femininity, blood, the bowl of sacred power and its connection to higher states of consciousness.
2. Acknowledge and honor that we are all connected, entangled, energy changing form.
3. Summon the spiritual, emotional and physical body's awareness.
4. Summon the Goddess, the most feminine essence of you.

Imagery

- Imagine women sitting together in a sacred circle, representing the sacred void, the period, creation, the universe within and without, as above, so below, honoring the sacred portal to transport spirit into a human body.
- The bowl of sacred power pulls up the earth energies, known as the Dragon lines or Lei lines, through our gateway, the portal. Mother Earth infuses us with primordial energy, clarity, and ancient wisdom as her frequency guides our true steps in power, balance and harmony with nature.
- Look up and honor the magnetics of the moon, reaching up and pulling her down and into the bowl of sacred power: dark moon we bleed, crescent moon we ovulate, full moon we shine.
- We feel our body's primordial fluid tides ebb and flow with the fullness of the moon, awakening our dream.
- Honor our connections to all things seen and unseen; the dimensional portal, womb consciousness that transfers, transports and transcends.

You've finished. Before you go…

Tweet/share that you finished this book.

Please star rate this book.

Reviews are solid gold to writers. Please take a few minutes to give us some itty bitty feedback.

ABOUT THE AUTHOR

In 1954 when I had my first period at age 11, it was minimally discussed and at first, I thought something was very wrong with me. There was no ritual, no celebration and it was hidden like a secret; a stigma of "that time of the month" or "the curse". Every month I hid it and was afraid that anyone, would know that I was menstruating.

In 1966, I delivered my daughter Heather two weeks early by breach vaginal birth; both of us could have died. At that time, just the doctor and nurse were present. My husband and family members were not waiting in the hospital for us; those were ignorant times.

In March 1994, I was called unexpectedly and within 24 hours arrived in the jungle in Mexico. Through this adventure, life as I knew it changed forever. As I wrote Spiritual Energy 13, I was reminded that this journey opened the gateway to universal awareness.

In 1995, at age 52, I was diagnosed with uterine cancer. The body is the great teacher that can bring you to your knees. The body says, "When you learn about me you learn about the universe", for within you is a universe by divine design as mysterious as consciousness. Rhona Jordan, the grandmother, the crone, offers this book in celebration of a woman's bowl of sacred power and to shout that it is – **O.K. to talk about it!**

Other Amazing Itty Bitty Books

- **Your Amazing Itty Bitty® Imagery Book**
  – Rhona Jordan, C.GIt., C.CHt.

- **Your Amazing Itty Bitty® Meditation Book**
  – Rhona Jordan, C.GIt., C.CHt.

- **Your Amazing Itty Bitty® Interstitial Cystitis Book**
  – Rhona Jordan, C.GIt., C.CHt.

- **Your Amazing Itty Bitty® Physics of Consciousness Book**
  – Rhona Jordan, C.GIt., C.CHt.

With many more Amazing Itty Bitty® books available online…

www.ingramcontent.com/pod-product-compliance
Lightning Source LLC
Chambersburg PA
CBHW061305040426
42444CB00010B/2523